The Pregnancy Cookbook

25 Quick & Easy Recipes packed with the Nutrients needed During Pregnancy

Thomas Kelley

INTRODUCTION

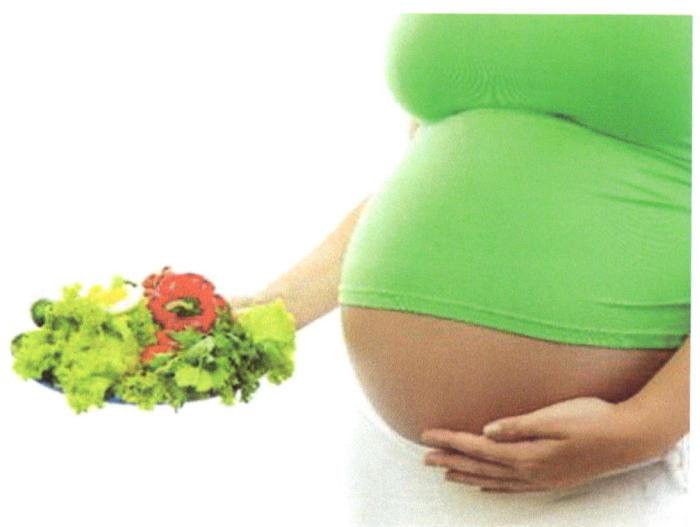

It is important that every expecting mother understands that everything that goes into her body can affect the baby that is currently developing inside her. Unfortunately energy and time are often a commodity that mothers-to-be just don't have and it is these two very commodities that are often needed when trying to eat right. This, my friend, is where the book '*25 Quick & Easy Recipes packed with the Nutrients needed During Pregnancy*' comes in as it is packed with amazing recipes that are quick and easy to make while still providing all the required nutrients for your baby to remain safe and healthy.

Here are 25 quick, easy and healthy recipes that all expecting mothers can enjoy with their whole family regardless of the mood they may be in. The recipes are divided into 4 categories; breakfast, lunch, dinner and snacks so you will have the perfect meal regardless of the time of day. All the recipes in this book will contain essential nutrients for you and baby. These include

- Protein: Expecting mothers need a minimum of 80g of protein daily to help the formation of your developing baby.
- Complex Carbohydrates: These are the foods that will provide the required fiber and other vitamins and nutrients keep your digestive system running smoothly as well as aid in the bone development and to prevent birth defects and anemia in your growing fetus. This food group will also help in getting you energy and ease morning sickness.
- Healthy Fats: These foods help in the brain and eye development of your baby and reduces the event of inflammation for the mother. They can also aid in the prevention of depression (whether prenatal or post-partum) and early labor. These are also the foods that will increase the production of breast milk.

All of these nutrients combined with your necessary supplements and vitamins will ensure a healthy and safe delivery of your little bundle of joy. So without further ado let's dive in, shall we?

TABLE OF CONTENTS

INTRODUCTION.. 2

BREAKFAST 6

SPINACH SMOOTHIE 7

PB&J OATMEAL 9

EGG MUFFINS 11

SWEET POTATO HASH 13

SOUTHWESTERN SCRAMBLE 15

COOKIE DOUGH CEREAL 17

LUNCH 19

WHOLE WHEAT PITA SANDWICH...................................... 20

SUPER FOOD SALAD.. 22

BURRITO BOWL 24

TURKEY BURGER 26

VEGGIE PIZZA.. 28

TACO SALAD 30

DINNER 32

BAKED SALMON AND GREENS 33

SPINACH, STRAWBERRY, AND CHICKEN SALAD 35

SHRIMP & VEGETABLE ROAST 37

SNACKS 39

APPLE ALMOND SANDWICHES 40

VEG AND DIP 42

GRAPE KEBABS 44

BLUEBERRY & MARSHMALLOW KEBABS 46

CUCUMBER SALAD 48

CLEMENTINE IN CINNAMON SYRUP 50

SUGAR SNAP AND CHEESE DIP 52

CHERRY TOMATOES AND CHEESE DIP 54

CRAB STUFFED AVOCADO 56

TEXAS CAVIAR 58

BREAKFAST

BREAKFAST IS THE MOST IMPORTANT MEAL OF THE DAY AS IT SETS IN THE ENERGY LEVELS FOR THE WHOLE DAY. FOR PREGNANT LADIES THIS IS EVEN MORE ESSENTIAL AS YOU WILL WANT TO START THE DAY RIGHT AND TO KEEP YOUR MORNING SICKNESS UNDER CONTROL.

SPINACH SMOOTHIE

Break should be fun, easy and delicious! So, here is a quick and easy recipe that contains all the required nutrients in one cup. This is perfect if you are often riddled with annoying morning sickness.

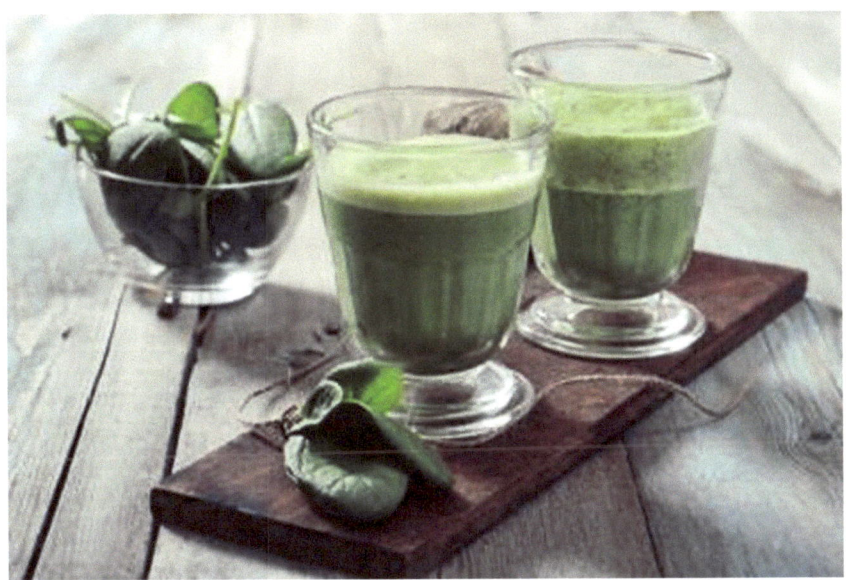

Yields: 1 Glass

Time Needed: 7 minutes

INGREDIENTS:

- Greek Yogurt (Non-fat, ½ cup)
- Spinach (1 handful, cut up into pieces)
- Frozen Fruit (any fruit of your choice, 1 cup, chopped)
- Flaxseed (2 tbsp.)
- Water (just a little, about 4ozs.)

DIRECTIONS:

1. Simply pour all the ingredients into a blender, pour it in a cup and enjoy.

PB&J Oatmeal

Quick, easy and nutritious!

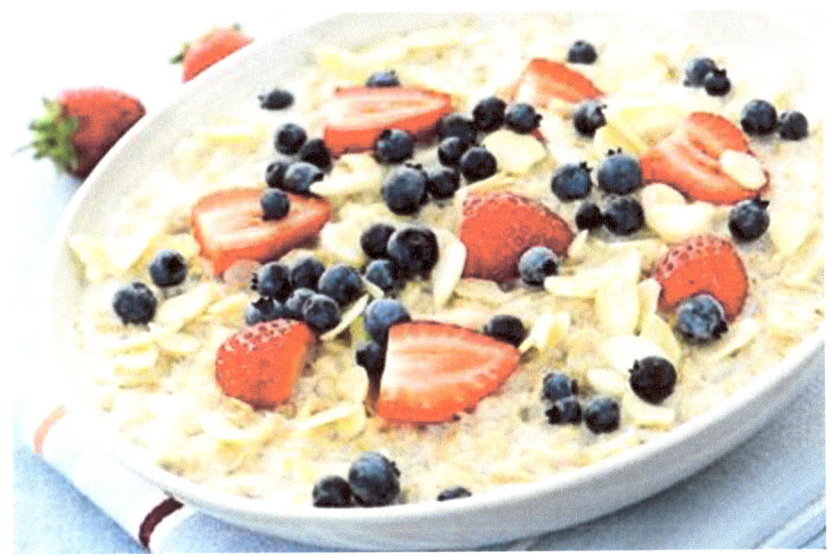

Yields: 1 serving

Time Needed: 10 minutes

INGREDIENTS:

- Old Fashion Oats (1/2 cup, rolled)
- Blueberries (1/2 cup, frozen)
- Peanut Butter (1 tbsp.)

DIRECTIONS:

1. Using the directions on the box, make about ½ cup of oatmeal.
2. Mix in the peanut butter and blueberries.
3. Serve and enjoy.

EGG MUFFINS

That's right! You can have delicious egg muffins for a protein blast in the morning.

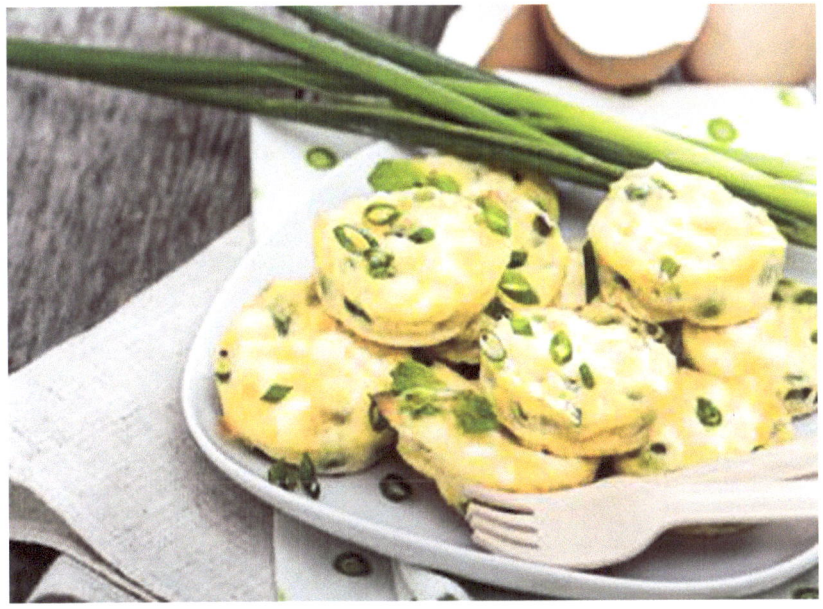

Yields: 6 Muffins

Time Needed: 30 minutes

INGREDIENTS:

- Eggs (6, large)
- Lean Meat (any on your choice, 6 slices)
- Veggies (any of your choice, chopped)

DIRECTIONS:

1. Set your oven to preheat at 350 degrees.
2. Whisk your 6 eggs in a large bowl.
3. Prepare a non-stick muffin pan and add your lean meat to each cup.
4. Pour in your chopped veggies evenly in the 6 molds and top off by pouring in your whisked egg evenly in all 6 molds.
5. Bake until browned (should be about 20 minutes)
6. Cool, serve and enjoy.

Sweet Potato Hash

Easy and filling meal packed with the essential nutrients needed for pregnancy.

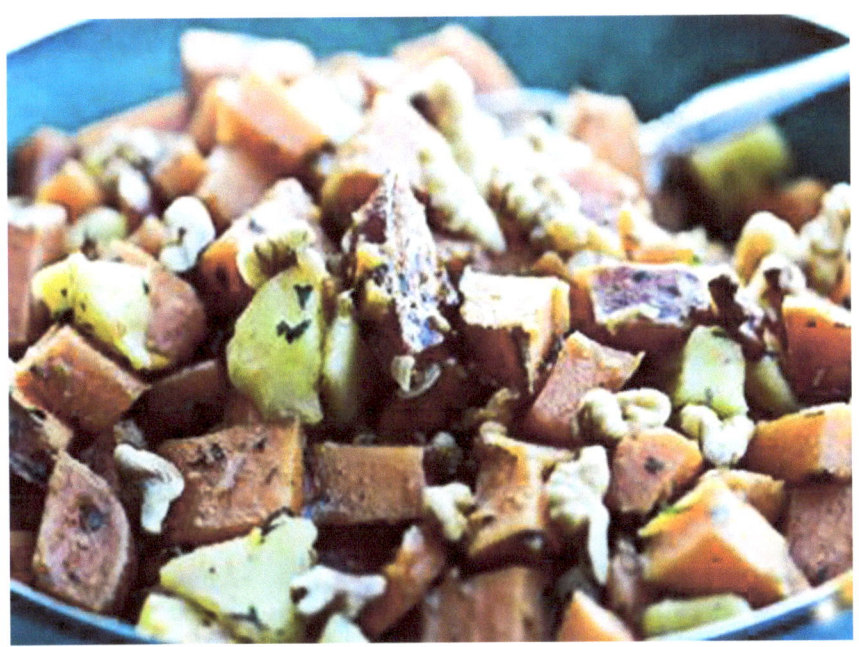

Serves: 2

Total Time Needed: 20 minutes

INGREDIENTS:

- Eggs (2 large, scrambled)
- Lean Meat (of your choice)
- Vegetables (Chopped)
- Sweet Potatoes (chopped)

DIRECTIONS:

1. Prepare a large greased skillet over medium heat.
2. Proceed to scrambling eggs, add in the vegetables, sausage and lean meat
3. Finally add your sweet potato.
4. Serve and Enjoy!

SOUTHWESTERN SCRAMBLE

Who says eggs has to be boring? Get a vibrant, healthy and colorful meal in minutes.

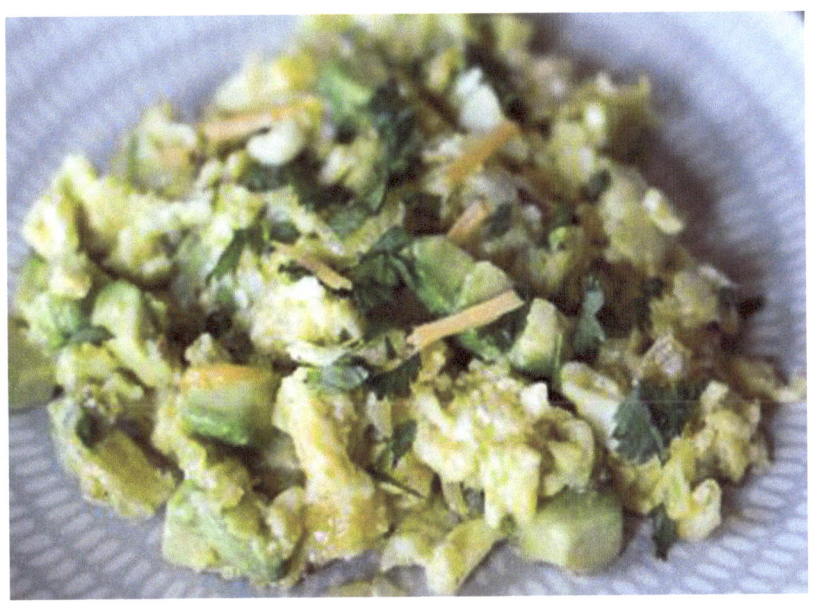

Image Credit: Flickr user Mallydally,
<https://www.flickr.com/photos/39975765@N05/8717329080/sizes/l >

Serves: 2

Time Needed: 15 minutes

INGREDIENTS:

- Eggs (2, large)
- Chiles (2 small, hatch, chopped)
- Green Onion (1, chopped)
- Chicken (1 breast, shredded)
- Avocado (1/2, chopped)
- Butter (1 tsp)

DIRECTIONS:

1. Whip eggs in a small container while your skillet heats on the fire.
2. Add butter to the hot pan and spread so that the entire pan is greased.
3. Pour in your whipped eggs, chicken, chopped onion, avocado pieces and chiles and mix well until eggs are evenly scrambled.
4. Serve and Enjoy!

COOKIE DOUGH CEREAL

Cereal just isn't the same without some cookie dough and chocolate chips.

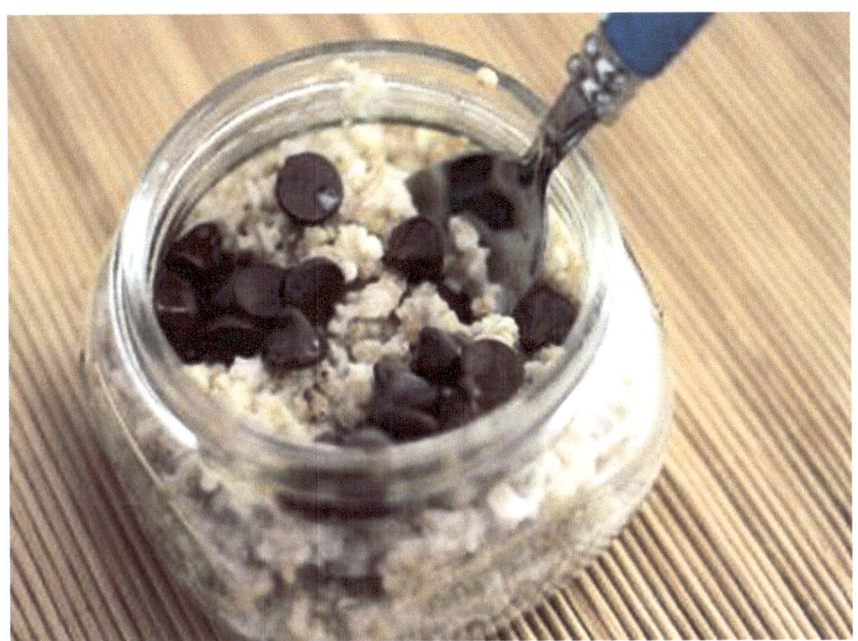

Image Credit: Flickr user StarsApart,
<https://www.flickr.com/photos/meginsanity/5777093323/sizes/l>

Serves: 1

Total Time Needed: 10 minutes

INGREDIENTS:

- Rolled Oats (old fashioned, ½ cup)
- Peanut Butter (2 tbsp.)
- Honey (1 tsp.)
- Chocolate Chips (unsweetened)
- Milk (½ cup)

DIRECTIONS:

1. In a small bowl mix all the ingredients, except your milk and chocolate chips, together until crumbly.
2. Add your milk and chocolate chips.
3. Serve and Enjoy.

LUNCH

MID – DAY MEALS TO KEEP YOU ENERGIZED
UNTIL DINNER. ALL QUICK, EASY AND
DELICIOUS.

WHOLE WHEAT PITA SANDWICH

An easy sandwich that you can make that is nutritious for you while pregnancy.

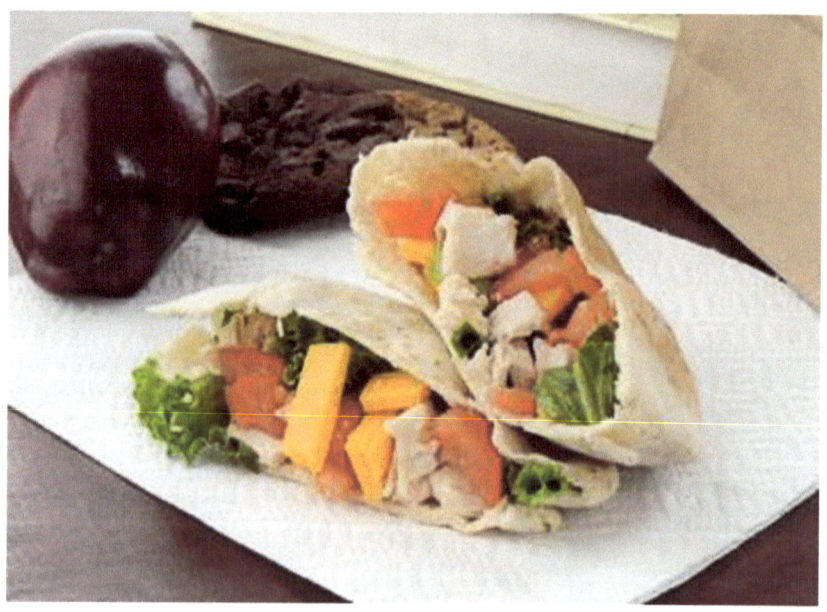

Serves: 2

Total Time Needed: 20 minutes

INGREDIENTS:

- Baby spinach
- Lean Meat (of your choice)
- Vegetables (Chopped)
- Goat cheese/ Spicy mustard
- Pita

DIRECTIONS:

1. Prepare a bowl that is big enough to add most of your ingredients.
2. Add the chopped vegetables, your lean meat, spicy mustard/goat cheese and the baby spinach into the bowl and stir well.
3. Stuff the ingredients from the bowl into the pita
4. Serve and enjoy

SUPER FOOD SALAD

An exciting that is packed with the essential nutrients needed for pregnancy.

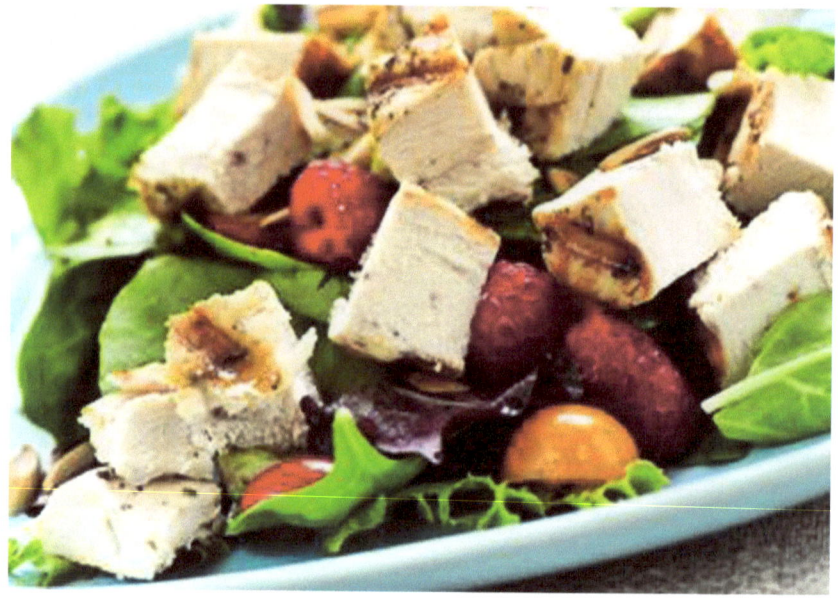

Serves: 2

Total Time Needed: 20 minutes

INGREDIENTS:

- Kale
- Nuts/Seed (one of your liking)
- Vegetables (Chopped)
- Berries
- Olive oil
- Apple cider vinegar
- Chicken (Grilled)
- Egg (hard-broiled)
- Lean meat (Your choosing)

DIRECTIONS:

1. Prepare the grill chicken and hardboiled egg beforehand.
2. Add the Kale, chopped veggies, nuts/seed, berries, olive oil and apple cider vinegar into bowl. Mix the ingredients well.
3. Serve all your ingredients and enjoy

BURRITO BOWL

Tasty, quick, easy and nutritious!

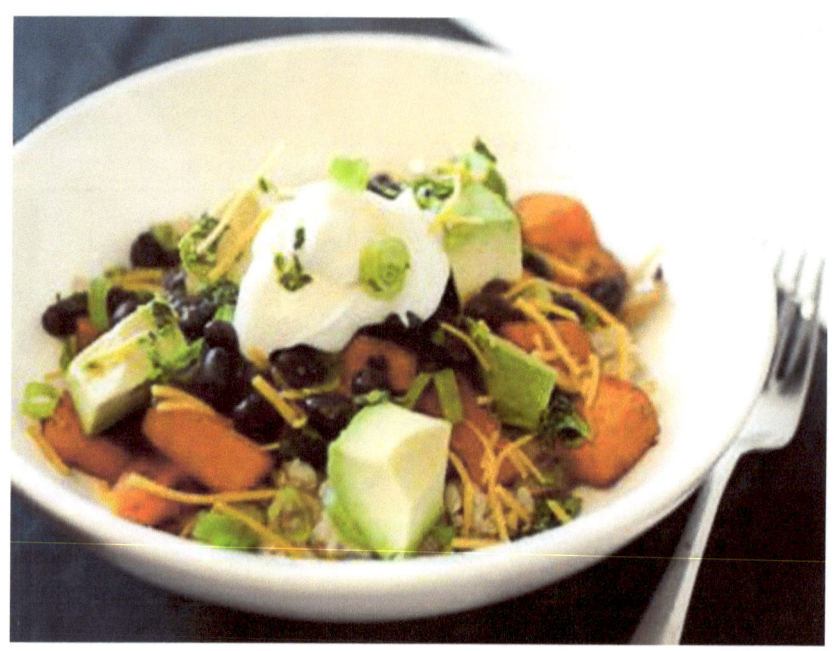

Image Credit: Flickr user Bobbi Bowers,
<https://www.flickr.com/photos/b_2/5631471286/>

Serves: 2

Total Time Needed: 20 minutes

INGREDIENTS:

- Cooked brown rice
- Roasted red peepers
- Black beans
- Roasted tomatoes
- Avocado
- Lime juice/Lime
- Lean meat (Your choosing)

DIRECTIONS:

1. Prepare the brown rice beforehand.
2. Add all the ingredients with the rice.
3. Stir well, serve and enjoy.

TURKEY BURGER

A pregnant woman should enjoy the finest burgers in life which pack with nutrients that is fit for a Queen.

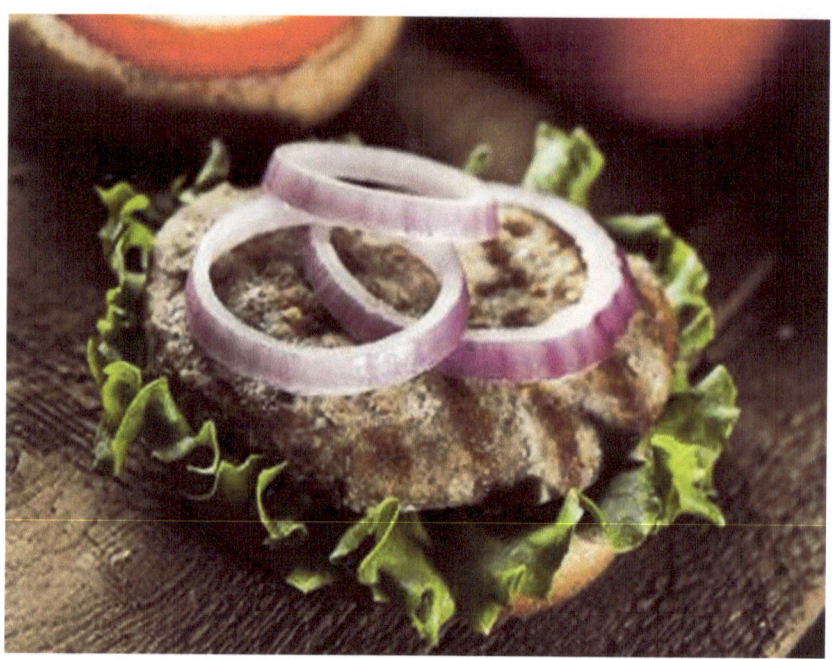

Serves: 2

Total Time Needed: 20 minutes

INGREDIENTS:

- Turkey breast (grounded)
- Tomato
- Spinach
- Onion
- Avocado
- Sweet Potatoes
- 1 teaspoon Grape seed oil

DIRECTIONS:

1. Your grounded turkey breast should and must mix your powder seasoning.
2. Use the meat to make a patty and grill the meat to your liking.
3. Cut the sweet potatoes into fries shape and put some grape seed oil on. Bake the fries to your liking.
4. Serve and enjoy.

VEGGIE PIZZA

Everyone one loves pizza. Here is a healthy pizza recipe

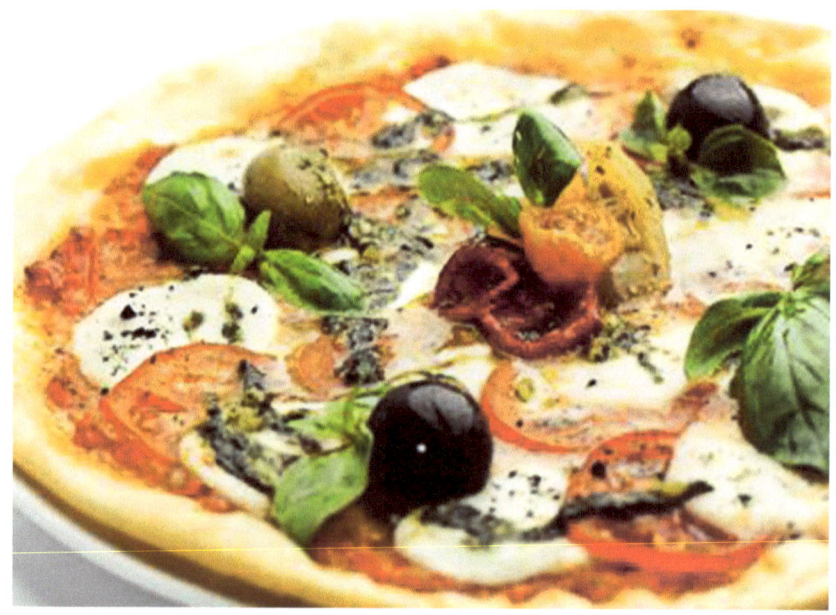

Serves: 2
Total Time Needed: 20 minutes

INGREDIENTS:

- Tomato
- Spinach
- Roasted red peeper
- Garlic
- Onion
- Avocado
- Whole wheat naan
- Chicken
- Mozzarella Cheese
- Basil (fresh)

DIRECTIONS:

1. Lay the whole wheat naan in a pizza dish.
2. Top it with all the remaining ingredients.
3. Place the dish in the oven and bake for 10 minutes.
4. Serve and enjoy.

TACO SALAD

A Taco salad for those Taco lovers.

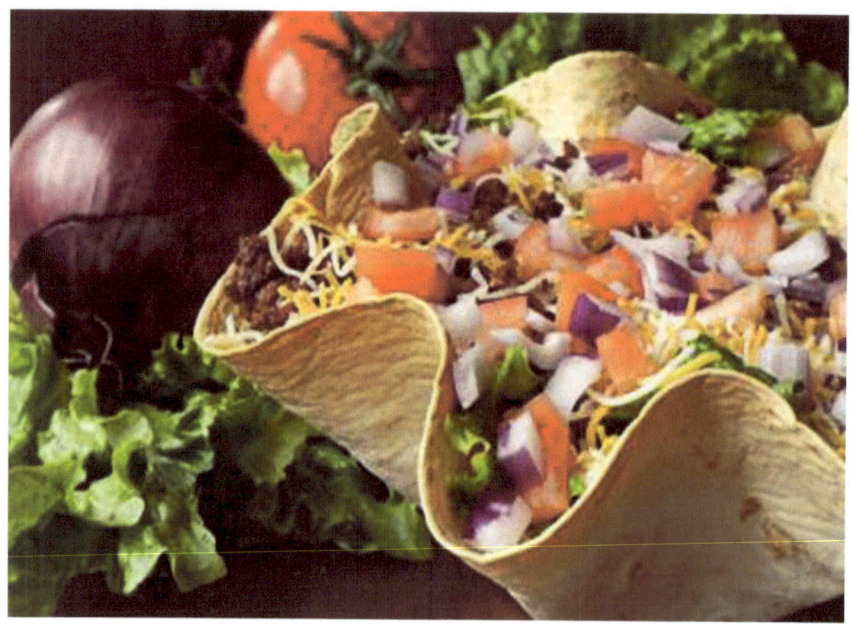

Serves: 2

Total Time Needed: 20 minutes

INGREDIENTS:

- Tortillas (Whole wheat)
- Olive oil
- Salt
- Romaine
- Grounded Beef
- Colby Jack Cheese
- Vegetables (chopped, any of your choice)
- Avocado (sliced)
- Greek yogurt

DIRECTIONS:

1. Make taco shells using whole wheat tortillas. Add some olive oil and some salt.
2. Place the shells in a safe bowl and put in the oven with a temperature of 400 degree for 10 minutes.
3. Top it with all the remaining ingredients.
4. Serve and enjoy.

DINNER

THE FINAL MEAL OF THE DAY! THIS
SECTION WILL LIST NUTRITION PACKED
MEALS THAT SHOULD BE USED TO END
YOUR DAY.

BAKED SALMON AND GREENS

It doesn't get healthier than baked fish and vegetables. It's delicious, easy to make and packed with nutrients.

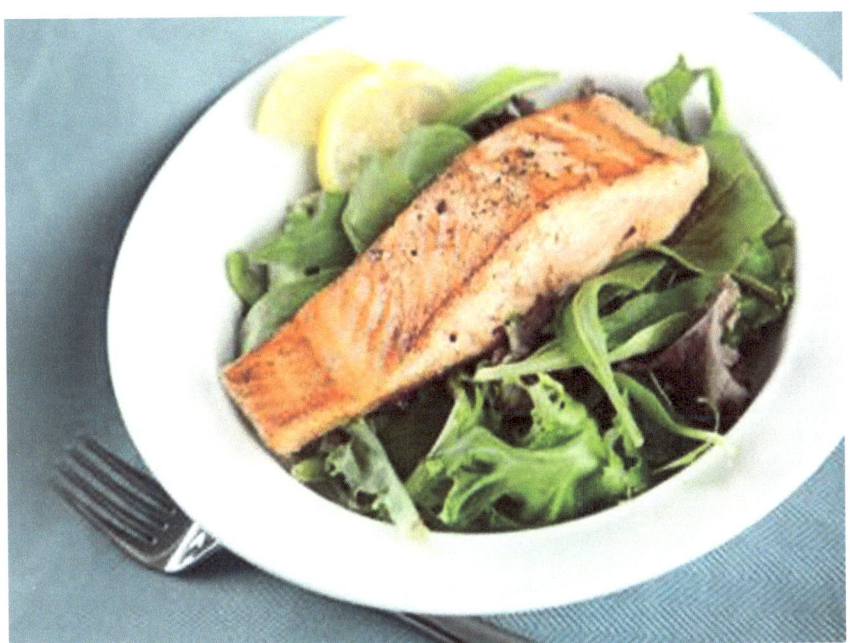

Serves: 2

Total Time Needed: 45 minutes

INGREDIENTS:

- Salmon fillets (2, ½ lb. cuts)
- Extra Virgin Olive Oil
- String Beans (½ lbs.)
- Tomatoes (1/2 , sliced)
- Green Onions (1, small, diced)
- Salt
- Pepper

DIRECTIONS:

1. Place your Oven to preheat at 350 degrees and Set a pot on water on the stove top to boil.
2. Place a piece of your salmon in a square of aluminum foil and top with some onion, tomato, salt, pepper, sprinkle with olive oil and fold then completely cover with foil.
3. Repeat step 2 for second fillet.
4. Place both fillets in the oven and allow to cook until tender and flaky (about 15 – 20 minutes)
5. Cut the stems from your string beans and place in your heated water and cook for about 5 minutes.
6. Remove from heat, serve and enjoy.

Spinach, Strawberry, and Chicken Salad

Here is a filling and tasty salad that will leave you wanting more.

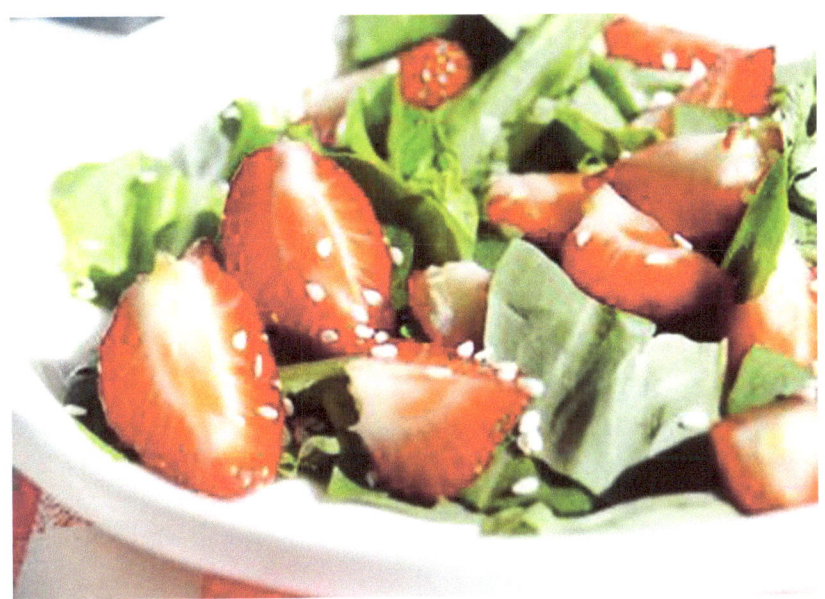

Serves: 2
Time Needed: 10 minutes

INGREDIENTS:

- Spinach (baby, 1 bundle)
- Strawberry (3 large, sliced)
- Almonds (as much as you desire, sliced)
- Cucumber (1 small, diced)
- Chicken (grilled slices)
- Vinaigrette (any you prefer

DIRECTIONS:

1. Add all the ingredients in a large bowl, while tossing, sprinkle with vinaigrette.
2. Serve and Enjoy.

SHRIMP & VEGETABLE ROAST

The perfect line between gourmet and comfort food. This is a recipe that you will have to make more than once.

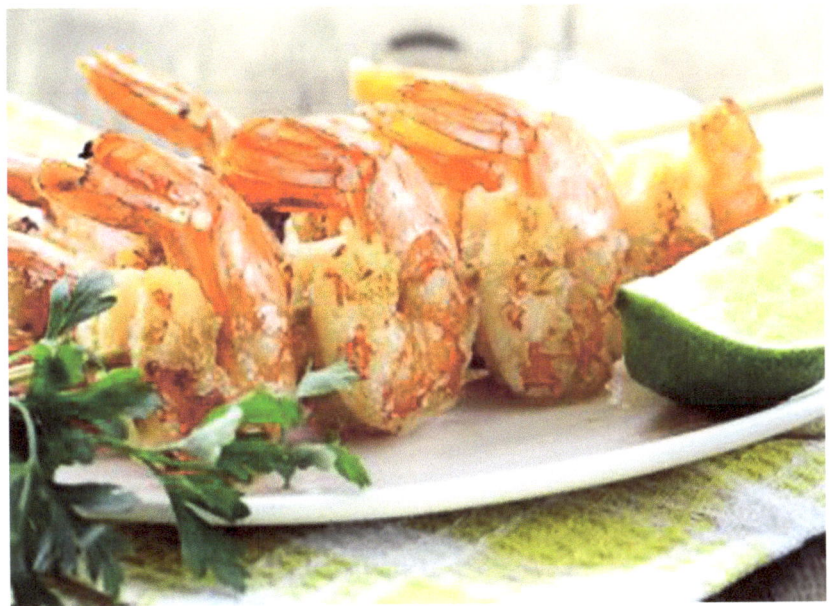

Serves:	3
Total Time Needed:	20 min

INGREDIENTS:

- Shrimp (Peeled, De-vined, Pre – cooked, pack of 12 medium)
- Garlic (2 cloves, minced)
- Cauliflower
- Onion (1 small, minced)
- Garlic (2 cloves, diced)
- Tomatoes (1 small, chopped)
- Olive Oil (1 tbsp.)
- Lemon Juice (1 tsp.)
- Salt (to taste)
- Pepper (to taste)

DIRECTIONS:

1. Set your oven to preheat at 350 degrees.
2. In a large bowl, toss all the ingredients together then transfer to a baking dish.
3. Cover with aluminum foil and place in the oven to roast until the vegetables have been cooked through and the shrimp turns pink.

SNACKS

LIGHT MEALS FOR ANY TIME OF THE DAY
TO FILL THAT EVER SO COMMON VOID!
THESE RECIPES WILL OFTEN BE A LIFESAVER
FOR YOU AS THEY OFTEN DON'T REQUIRE
YOU STEPPING IN ANY HEAT AND CAN BE
EATEN ON THE GO.

APPLE ALMOND SANDWICHES

Amazingly Easy and Delicious!

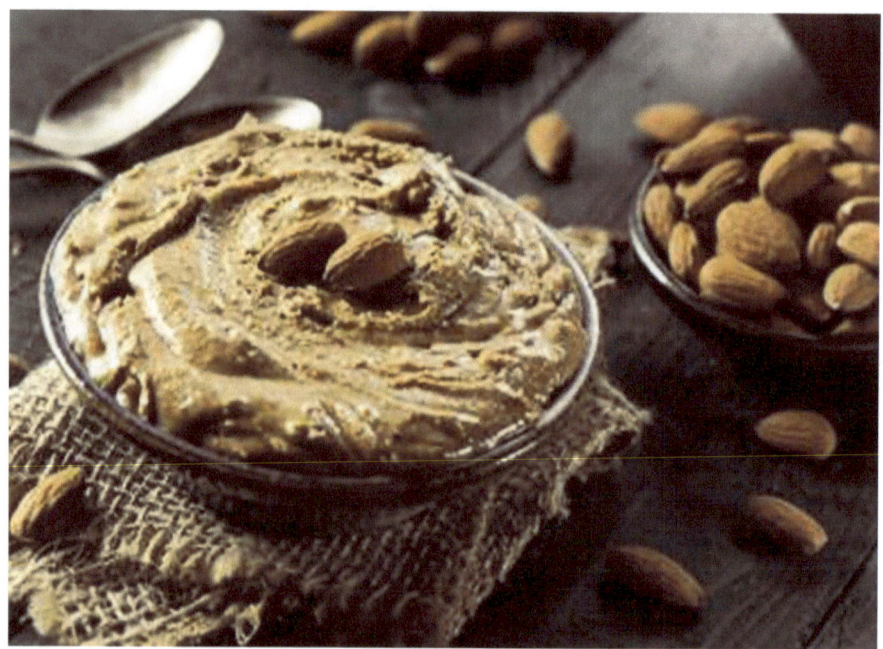

Serves: 2

Time Needed: 5 minutes

INGREDIENTS:

- Apple Slices (4 even slices)
- Almond Butter (for spreading)
- Chocolate Chips (unsweetened, as much as you like)

DIRECTIONS:

1. Spread your almond butter between two slices of apples sprinkle with chocolate chips,
2. Close to make a sandwich and repeat with the other 2 slices.
3. Serve and Enjoy!

VEG AND DIP

This is great for persons with a sweet tooth but doesn't want to go all out nuts on sugar.

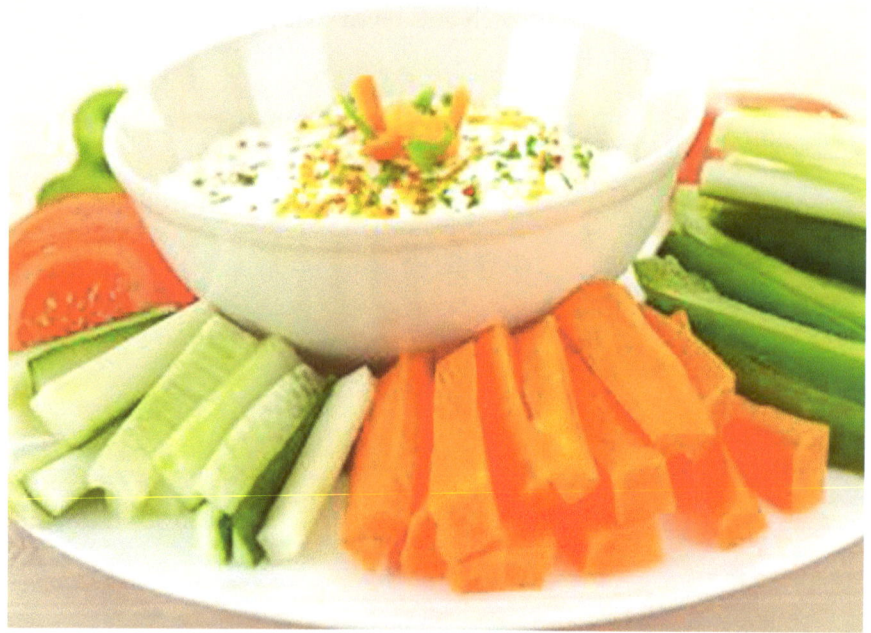

Serves: 4

Time Needed: 5 minutes

INGREDIENTS:

- Carrots (2 large, cut into strips)
- Celery (3 stalks, cut into pieces)
- Bell Peppers (about 3 large, cut into pieces)
- Cauliflower (¼ lb., cut into pieces)
- Yogurt (low fat, any flavor of your choice)

DIRECTIONS:

1. Pour your yogurt out into a small dipping container and set in the center of a platter.
2. Lay out the vegetable pieces around the dip.
3. Serve and Enjoy!

GRAPE KEBABS

Keeping a few of these in your refrigerator will prove to be a lifesaver in more ways than one,

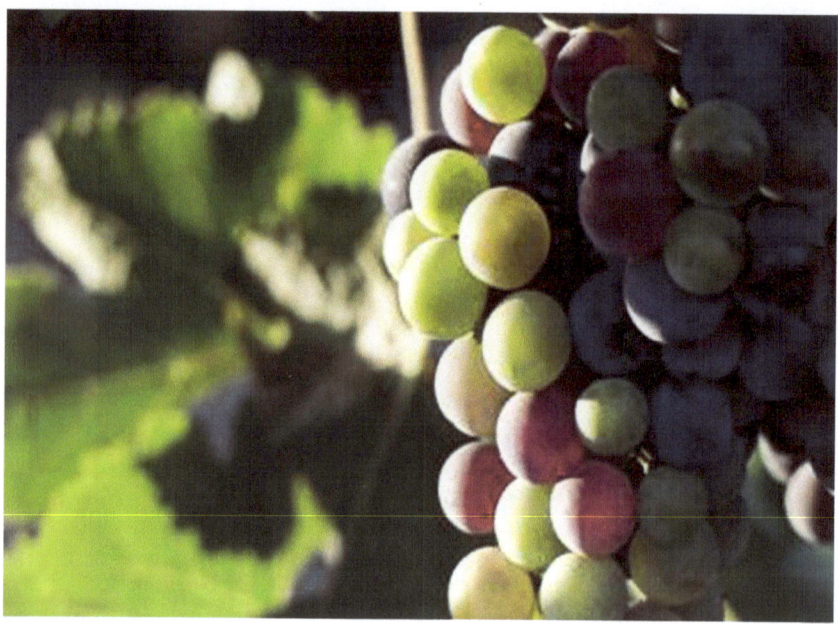

Serves: 3

Time Needed: 5 minutes

INGREDIENTS:

- Grapes (54 grapes of a different variety)

DIRECTIONS:

1. Using 9 kebab sticks, stick 6 grapes on each.
2. Store in the refrigerator until ready to eat.
3. Serve and Enjoy!

Blueberry & Marshmallow Kebabs

Let's make snack time interesting with blueberry and marshmallow kebabs.

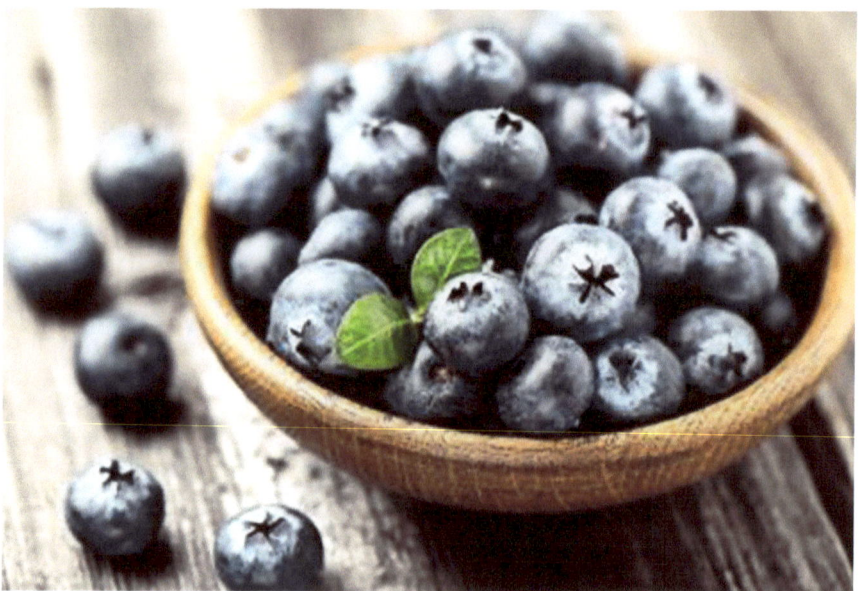

Serves: 3
Time Needed: 5 minutes

INGREDIENTS:

- Blueberries (27 small, cubed)
- Marshmallows (27, round)

DIRECTIONS:

1. Using 9 kebab sticks, stick 3 blueberries and marshmallows on each alternating both.
2. Store in the refrigerator until ready to eat.
3. Serve and Enjoy!

CUCUMBER SALAD

Nice, healthy and delicious!

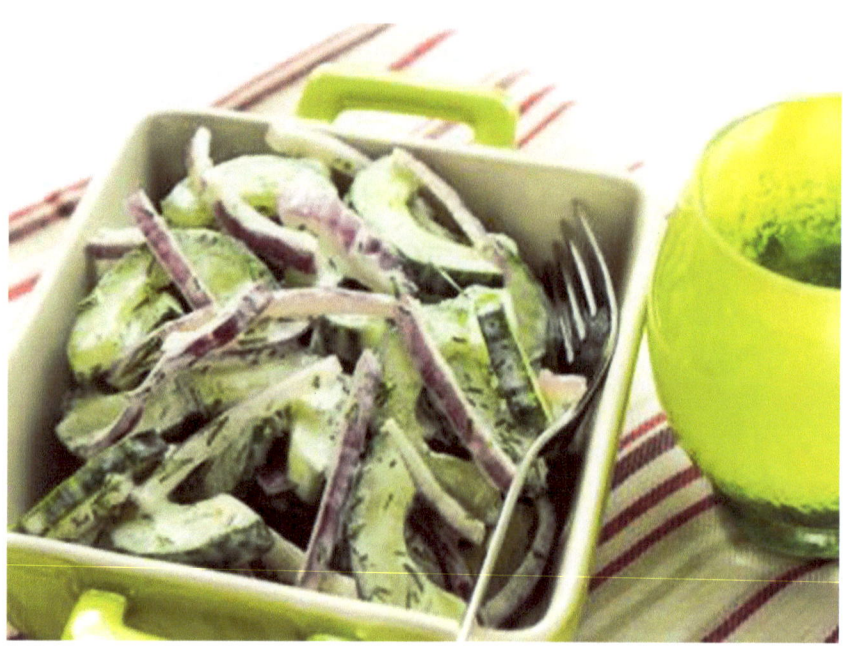

Serves: 1

Time Needed: 10 minutes

INGREDIENTS:

- Cucumber (1 medium, sliced)
- Yogurt (preferably Greek, 1 can)
- Vinegar (Apple Cider, 1 tbsp.)
- Onion (1, red, chopped)
- Dill (1 sprig, dried, only need leaves)
- Sugar (1 tsp)

DIRECTIONS:

1. Combine all the ingredients in a large bowl.
2. Toss until fully combined.
3. Serve and Enjoy.

CLEMENTINE IN CINNAMON SYRUP

A dash of citrus paired with a hint of cinnamon and you will be in heaven.

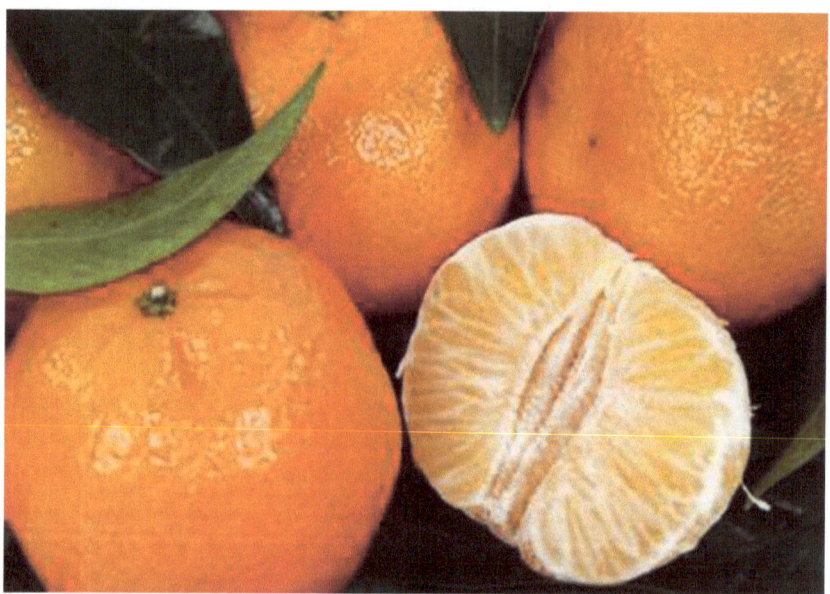

Serves: 3

Time Needed: 10 minutes

INGREDIENTS:

- Clementine (6 medium, sliced)
- Cinnamon Syrup (enough to cover your slices)

DIRECTIONS:

1. Slice your clementine and transfer to a medium sized mixing bowl.
2. Add your cinnamon syrup to the bowl until it just about covers the slices.
3. Allow to rest for 5 minutes, covered in the refrigerator.
4. Serve and Enjoy!

SUGAR SNAP AND CHEESE DIP

An easy snack packed with protein!

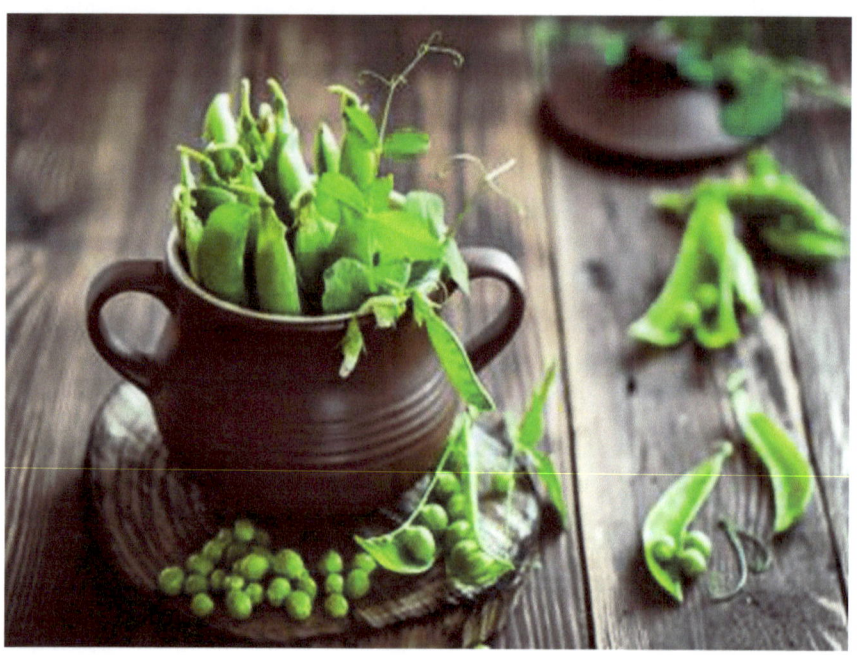

Serves: 1

Time Needed: 5 minutes

INGREDIENTS:

- Sugar Snap Peas (12, thoroughly washed)
- Goat Cheese (as much as you want)

DIRECTIONS:

1. Pour your goat cheese into a small dipping bowl and place in the center of a platter.
2. Spread you sugar snap peas around the platter.
3. Serve and Enjoy!

CHERRY TOMATOES AND CHEESE DIP

Tomatoes and cheese! What's better than that?

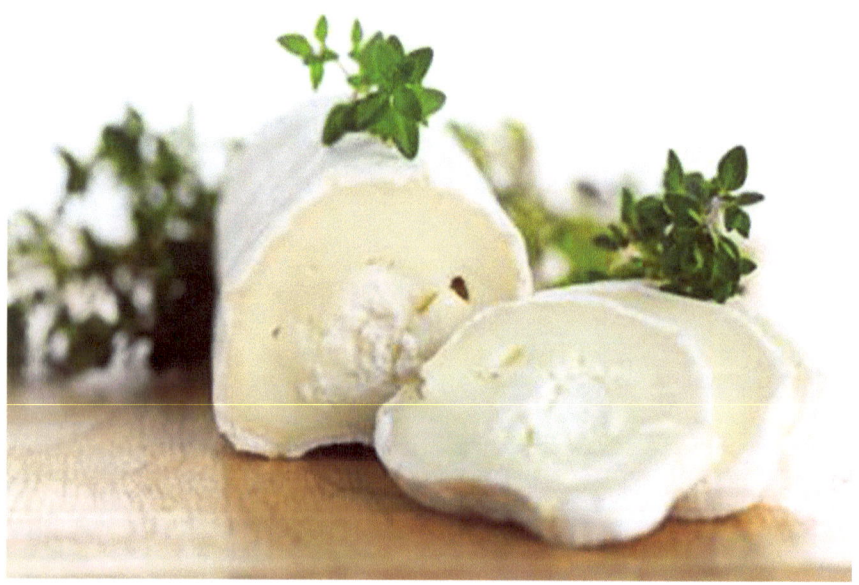

Serves: 1

Time Needed: 5 minutes

INGREDIENTS:

- Cherry Tomatoes (6, roasted)
- Warm Goat Cheese (as much as you want)

DIRECTIONS:

1. Pour your goat cheese into a platter.
2. Spread your tomato slices around the platter.
3. Serve and Enjoy!

CRAB STUFFED AVOCADO

Who says expecting mothers can't have seafood? Definitely not us and this recipe will prove to you why.

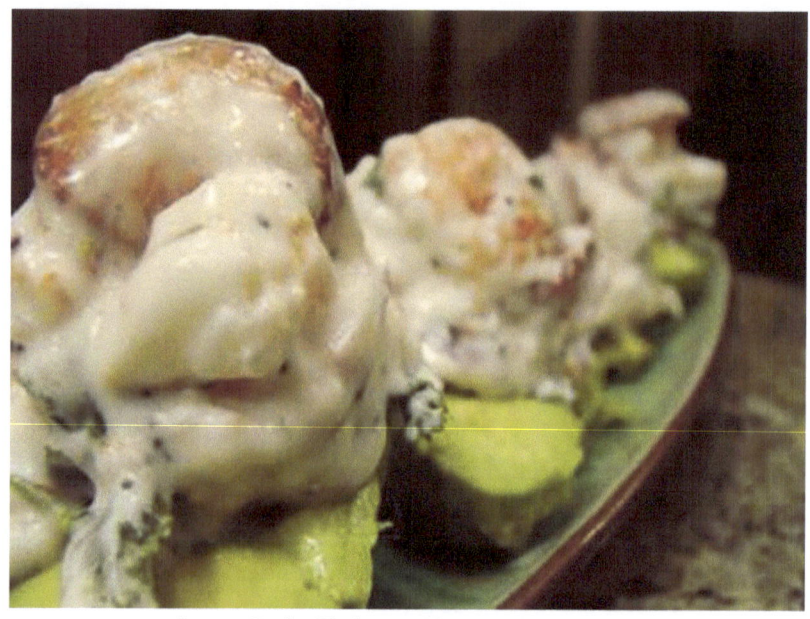

Image Credit: Flickr user Vegan Feast Catering,
<https://www.flickr.com/photos/veganfeast/3828354335/sizes/l>

Serves: 2

Time Needed: 10 minutes

INGREDIENTS:

- Avocado (1 large, halved)
- Crab Meat (precooked and seasoned)

DIRECTIONS:

1. Spoon your cooked crabmeat into your halves of avocado.
2. Serve and Enjoy.

TEXAS CAVIAR

Vibrant, easy and delicious!

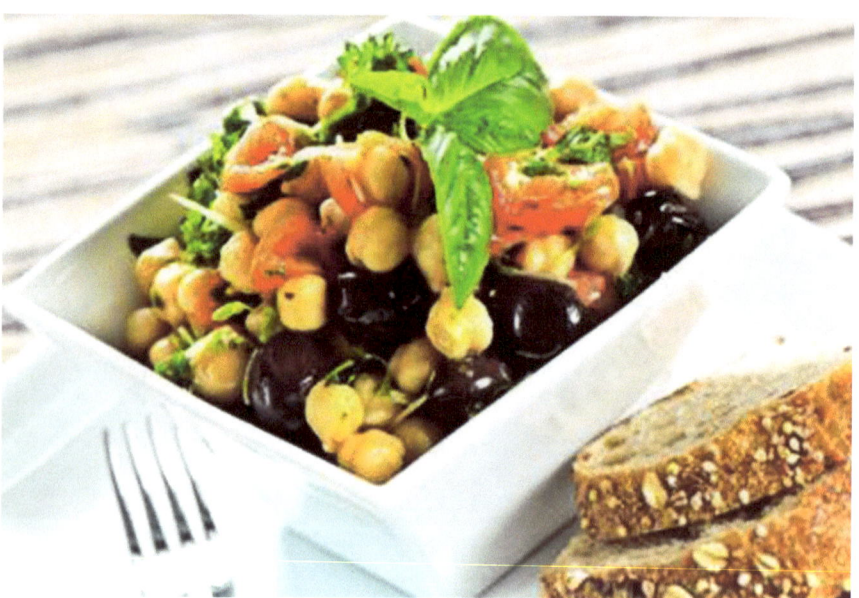

Serves: 4

Time Needed: 5 minutes

INGREDIENTS:

- Pinto Beans (½ lb.)
- Lime juice (1 tsp.)
- Cilantro (2 leaves)
- Pico de Gallo (½ lb.)
- Sweet Corn (½ lb.)

DIRECTIONS:

1. Toss ingredients together in a large bowl.
2. Serve and Enjoy!

www.ingramcontent.com/pod-product-compliance
Lightning Source LLC
Chambersburg PA
CBHW050823290526
45792CB00001B/232